Traditional and Modern Medicine: A Necessary Alliance

Why do we need a medical alliance?

Modern medicine relies heavily on treatments based on research that is scientifically approved and explainable. This eliminates traditional medicinal methods which use alternative and natural remedies for common illnesses. While the priority should be to treat ailments using whatever methods work, the notion that only pharmaceutical medicine can be prescribed begs the question: Has modern medicine become too modern?

Can western pharmaceutical medicine cure all diseases or ail the ailments? Or does it cause more side effects and long-term dependency on medication than helping the patient and curing the illness? Given that western medicine is only a recent event, is there any harm to engage in lateral thinking?

Modern or western medicine historically has a long list of accomplishments. Here are some of their notable achievements:

1882 Louis Pasteur discovered a method to prevent rabies.

1890 Emil von Behring, a German developed serum therapy and the diphtheria antitoxin as well as one for tetanus.

1895 Wiilhelm Conrad Rontgen produced and detected electromagnetic radiation discovering X-ray technology still used for scans.

1897 Chemists working in Germany producing the first aspirin.

1901 Karl Landsteiner identified different blood types and blood groups.

1901 Alois Alzheimer, a German psychiatrist identified Dementia and Alzheimer's disease

1903 Willem Einthoven, a Dutch doctor invented the ECG (electrocardiograph) machine.

1906 Sir Frederick Gowland Hopkins, an English biochemist discovered vitamin deficiencies and their role in causing scurvy and rickets.

1907 Paul Ehrichlich, a German doctor developed the treatment for syphilis

1921 Sir Frederick G Banting, a Canadian surgeon, discovered insulin

1923 Scientists discovered whooping cough, TB and tetanus injections.

1928 Alexander Flemming, a Scottish pharmacist invented penicillin using the growth of mould.

1929 Hans Berger, a German doctor discovered EEG (electroencephalography) which records brain activity.

1935 Max Theiler, a South African microbiologist started the dialysis machine and developed a vaccine against yellow fever.

1943 Wellem Koff built the first dialysis machine.

1946 Alfred Gilman and Louis Goodman pioneered cancer chemotherapy

1948 Julius Axelrod and Axlrod Brodie, two American chemists developed paracetamol.

1952 Jonas Salk, an American invents the polio vaccine

1953 John Gibbon, a surgeon develops the first successful heart-lung machine and performs the first case of cardiopulmonary bypass surgery.

1953 Inge Edler, a Swedish physician, invented echographs.

1959 Min Chueh Chang, a Chinese-American biologist developed the oral contraceptive pill and treatments in IVF

1960 Drs. Kouwenhoven, Safar, and Jude, a group of Americans develop cardiopulmonary resuscitation or CRP

1963 Leo Sternbach, a Polish chemist developed the first human lung transplant

1965 Dr Henry Meyer developed the first rubella vaccine

1966 Clarence Walton Lillehei pioneered Cardiothoracic surgery.

2020 Scientists develop the COVID -19 vaccination which is the largest modern-day breakthrough, saving the lives of millions worldwide

The Challenges We Face Today

While modern medicine continues to make headway, some significant challenges remain.

One is the upsurge of antibiotic resistance, partly in response to the overuse of antibiotics as well as pathogens and germs adapting to resist them. 30 years after the second World War, whereas there should be further research, breakthroughs and advancements, we instead face delays and bureaucracy which hinder diagnosis and treatment.

Millions of pounds were spent built hospitals without looking at the environmental impact of the design or the general health of the hospital and its staff. Instead, huge car parks were built out of consideration for visitors and patients (and revenue) causing stress and leading to more illnesses.

The journey from car park to the treatment room was not well-planned and patients with illnesses and accessibility needs have to walk through corridors, up and down stairs as well as use lifts causing unnecessary time delays and aggravation. This also does not take into consideration the mobility requirements of patients or their age. The appointment management system usually results in patients arriving then having to wait a considerable amount of time before they are called in to see someone. The patient may not have enough money to pay for the car park or they may face unreasonable delays due to the car park's location, leading to more problems.

Hospital environments also need a rehaul. Once a patient is admitted for surgery or an investigation, they should be discharged to a place conducive to healing. There are currently no gardens where they can breathe natural fresh air, sit on a bench and relax or lower their heart rate and blood pressure through natural plants and beauty.

Post-surgery, patients are sent back to the ward where they may be surrounded by other patients who could have complications and are offered substandard food which does not heal the body. An example is if a patient having just had a heart bypass returns to the ward and is offered on their food menu items full of fat such as pork, cheese or red meat. Beverages offered are full of sugar, caffeine or worse, artificial sweeteners and additives which cause more harm than good. Instead of colas and fizzy drinks, patients should receive water and fresh juices.

Agency staff in wards leads to a lack of continuous care for patients, especially when a nurse begins looking after a patient and a few hours later, another takes over unaware of their needs, temperament and comfort level.

There is also a lack of facilities and awareness for mental health in hospitals. Whereas counselling services operate, there are no proper procedures in place patients with manic or severe depression, schizophrenia, borderline personality disorder or those with suicidal tendencies. A system needs to be implemented where patients can be seen swiftly, particularly those who are deemed to be at high risk of self-harm. Due to COVID, many nurses doctors and other front like staff now suffer from post-traumatic stress disorder due to either losing loved ones, their own illnesses or because of their hospital experiences under immense pressure during the pandemic. Some are often depressed and need immediate attention. One year on from the pandemic, nothing has been done to address their needs which will lead to severe repercussions as their condition could become chronic.

It is also sad to see super specialties emerging like mushrooms. This is not good for patients or the medical industry. Specialists have become so specific that after a short time within there area of practice, they are unable to treat or diagnose anything other than the area they've qualified in, knowing too little about other parts of the body. This leads to more referrals for unnecessary complaints which would be best dealt with through a general physician's expertise. The specialists often do not take nor have the time to explain conditions and treatments with patients properly and with compassion. This is being observed among patients with cancer and even those who are terminally ill. The patients' families are also left with many unanswered questions and pastoral care is eroding at a fast rate.

Patients with multiple medical conditions are referred to a number of super specialists, with each one prescribing multiple prescriptions for each of their areas of treatment. This can not only lead to unwanted side effects and a non-holistic view of the condition but also cause confusion due to the timing of when to take medication. If one is to be taken in the morning and another three times a day, then another is a sleeping tablet, it risks a chemical cocktail that plays havoc with a person's wellbeing and routines. An elderly patient living on their own would now be at risk of taking an overdose or missing doses due to the many medications they have been prescribed. A patient with three medical complaints may end up taking nine forms of medication with others prescribed to counter side-effects from these. If a statin is prescribed for high cholesterol and its main side effect is severe muscular pain, then a super specialist may prescribe a morphine based painkiller to counter this. This is despite the specialist trying to help the patient! I would advise all patients to read their medication's information enclosed within its leaflet which details dosage, side effects and what to watch for if taking multiple medications.

The most important aspect of health is simply to be fit and healthy. Within the current system of medicine, lifestyle is often sidelined in favour of medication. If a patient is diabetic, the endocrinologist will only talk to them about cutting down on carbohydrates. In the case of a coronary heart condition, they will be advised only to cut down on fats. There is no holistic treatment which advises them to walk with details on how frequently, at which pace and where. A common complaint from patients is that they are told to walk more but not told in which manner so their manner of walking has no beneficial effect on their condition.

Those living in congested areas or near busy road may walk locally and be exposed to toxins, particulates and dust, which could make them worse or cause further sickness and respiratory problems. Some are advised to get more active and take up jogging, which causes wear and tear of the joints leading to the onset of osteoarthritis in the knees. Others join fitness centres and spend a fortune on memberships, ending up with overexertion, sprains, multiple joint issues and cartilage damage. The worst is the lack of decent air quality and ventilation. This leads to a person inhaling carbon dioxide expelled by others in the same room, which spreads airborne viruses and conditions. Due to the frequent cold weather, many buildings lack fresh air, proper ventilation and even windows.

Within recent years, American flooded the world with fast food and nutrition-poor choices such as Coca-Cola, Kentucky Fried Chicken and Starbucks. Many of our youth and even those in their twenties and thirties are addicted to Coca-Cola, indulge in cheap fast food such as McDonald's and fried chicken leading to high cholesterol, or drink too much Starbucks coffee as part of their lifestyle which is cardio toxic. Children are targeted from a young age with free toys with meals and fast food joints opening up within short distances of schools, as well as the common occurrence now of children's parties at places like McDonald's.

At present, the wealthy and powerful pharmaceutical industry controls with lobbying strength. They send medical representatives to see doctors from hospitals as well as in the community and influence them with perks. Even local councils approve the accumulation of takeaways and fast food shops around schools as these places commit to financially contribute to clean up of the local area or sponsor local sporting events. This is causing a lot of problems within communities and the nation's health is suffering from earlier ages because of it.

In some of the countries such as Great Britain, alternative medicines are banned in hospitals as well as in the community, justified with the argument that it is not evidence based!

Why can't we form an alliance between Traditional and Modern Medicine?

Seventy-five percent of the world is already using both traditional medicine and modern medicine. America, the world's wealthiest country, is a prime example. Most alternative medicines and minerals are readily available in pharmacies and supermarkets, yoga and meditation centres are full across the country and reflexologists, acupuncturists and herbalists have regular clients that remain with them for years. Osteopaths are as popular as the doctors and can prescribe medication and carry out investigations. In short, they are already undertaking an integrated approach to medicine. Local pharmacists can also offer advice and alternative treatment is cheap enough to be affordable to all.

There are at least five Ayurvedic colleges in America, who not only teach Ayurveda but are also making Ayurvedic medicines according to the principle of an integrated approach.

India, the world's most populated country, has widely used Ayurveda, Homeopathy and other herbal medications for decades. Ayurveda is over 5000 years old and is proven and time tested. All the medications are natural and not synthetic. Yoga, meditations and massages are all a part of Ayurveda. The management of Ayurveda was written by Charaka expanding to 5 volumes that explain all aspects of the human body and mind, advising how to keep healthy, how a treatment hospital should as well as socially conscious advice such as how or with whom you can have alcohol with. There are also details about performing surgery – and this was written 5000 years ago! This would indicate that the procedure of surgery existed before we formally recognized it.

Like India, China is a densely populated country and for centuries only used one system: Acupuncture. They have used western medications but integrated it into their system applying acupuncture procedures during major operations instead of anesthesia.

We also have Homeopathy. This wonderful treatment method is even effective for babies and small children with remedies for everything from teething and colds to coughs and fever-inducing conditions. Treatment is in the form of drops, pills and soft tablets that work within a minute and avoid febrile convulsion. Homeopathic remedies can also help with mental shock and bereavement-related issues.

There are, of course, instances when one must seek emergency assistance. If someone is having difficulty breathing, is unconscious or experiencing fits or chest pains, then there is no sense in contacting an acupuncturist! Only an emergency ambulance will do in these situations.

A problem with allopathic doctors is that after passing their exams, undertaking training and gaining practice, they think this is all there is to learn about medicine. Like a jockey riding a horse, they only look ahead as if the horse's side is protected by a shield. Tunnel vision is a curse for modern medicine and is unacceptable. We live in the real world and doctors take the Hippocratic oath, which is one of the toehold binding oaths of history. Written in antiquity, its principles are held sacred by doctors to this day, to treat the sick to the best of one's ability, preserve patient privacy, teach the secrets of medicine to the next generation and so on.

Doctors can learn from their patients and their beliefs too. It is a practitioner's duty to continue their training in their spare time and try to understand how alternative medicine works and can benefit society. One can read about their benefits in volumes of books in the local library without embarrassment and once understood, it can be put into practice.

The patients are innocent. If you cannot understand them, they will not benefit from your services. If you take the time to know them and their conditions, you will inevitably respect them more and serve them better. If you are still unclear about their condition in relation to their lifestyle, you can seek advice from local alternative clinics.

It is high time for medical schools to undergo reform and adopt these methods, ensuring everyone has the knowledge, training and practice required to best treat a patient.

We are also facing an increase in pollution and environmental hazards, which has led to more illnesses and excess deaths. While the 20th century saw a massive number of fatalities from infections, future centuries could also see that number rise even further.

Now is not yet time to sit back and relax.

The disappearing craft of medicine

The lack of time being dedicated to patients for consultation by doctors can be frustrating. The rise in the bureaucracy and necessary box-ticking exercises in addition to an increasingly older population with complex needs have all put pressure on the system and resulted in less time allocated for quality care. Ironically, patient care and to help humanity are the primary reasons the majority of medical professionals choose medicine as a profession, yet we are failing the patients catastrophically. Not enough time is dedicated to listening to patients and assessing their conditions as this has been replaced with the business, financial and political requirements of the practice. This contributes to the loss of accuracy, craft and teamwork which the patients expect and rely on from their doctor.

Experienced clinicians are now having to complete paperwork that hinders their work and prevents them from making the most of what they have learned over the years. Being overwhelmed by guidelines can prevent doctors using intuitive skills, which is a crucial component of patient care.

The changes have eliminated teamwork and severed the link between the nurses, health visitors and midwives.

Homeopathy

In homeopathic medicine it is assumed that there are three parts to the human being. These are the physical body, the mind and also the person themself. This is a system of therapeutics for treating people and animals on the basis of a simple principle. The word homeopathy is derived from the Greek words 'homoios' which means similar and 'pathos' meaning suffering.

Similia similibus curentur
Let likes be treated by likes.

In conventional medicine we are taught to think in terms of disease or pathological states and changes from the normal physiological state as a result of outside factors, such as infection, trauma or stress. In order to treat such diseased states, we try to make a diagnosis based on the symptoms and physical signs. As a result, the medicine becomes increasingly fragmented and specialised with only a few treatments which cure the patient as a whole.
According to Homeopathy, a patient's history is noted, using the Materia Medica. The root cause is treated as opposed to modern medicine which now mostly addresses the symptoms.

Batch flower remedies

Dr Edward Batch was a physician and a homoeopath, who spent his life searching for the purest methods of healing. He believed that the attitude of the mind plays a vital role in maintaining health and recovering from illness. He developed a complete system of 38 flower remedies from wild plants, trees or bushes.

The purpose of the remedies is to support the patient's fight against illness by addressing anxiety, depression, mental trauma and other emotional factors thought to impede physical healing.

"Health is our heritage, our right it is the complete and full union between soul, mind and body"
-Dr Edward Batch.

Acupuncture

The ancient Chinese described the flow of nervous energy in the body as 'Qi'- the energy of life. They believed it permeated everything and linked their surroundings together. In medicine, it is recognised as a wave of electrical depolarisation spreading along the nerve. The Chinese called the principal nerve endings 'acupuncture points' and the main course of a similar group of nerve endings 'meridians'. The aim of Chinese doctors is to correct the imbalance of the vital forces of the body. Once the harmonious interplay of these forces has been restored, the patient is able to overcome the effects of the illness.
In the organism, as everywhere else in nature an in the universe, there are two states of energy, yang and yin. Yang relates to sensitivity, tonicity, heat, dryness, light and the day. Yin is related to inactivity, atony, cold, humidity, shadow, the night and dark energy. The two states are opposing to each other and antagonists. The excess of one results in the dearth of the other and vice versa. A condition of health demands equilibrium between yang and yin. Imbalance with a clear predominance one or the other result in diseases.

The diagnosis of the yang and yin is through examination and interpretation of the pulses according to Chinese medicinal principles . Acupuncture does not create energy but can correct and neutralise its disturbance.

Treatments are carried out using acupuncture needles, massage and moxibustion.

Tai Chi

The ancient art of Tai Chi is dates back to over 5000 years ago. It focuses on balancing the energies in the body for optimum health and wellbeing. It can reduce the risk of falls in the elderly and also help with balance disorders . It is of particular benefit to the elderly who suffer from brittle bone disease. It can help to reduce high blood pressure levels and arthritis pain. Tai Chi is a series of slow-moving, meditative martial arts focused on balancing Yin and Yang through hand and body co-ordinated movements. It can also help develop physical strength and mobility as well as provide mental relaxation and improve breathing techniques.

Vastu Shastra and Feng Shui

Energy is all around us and in every place. There is a difference in the quality of energies that surrounds any living or workplace. By using Vastu Shastra or Feng Shui, one can create a favourable energy around any environment to help improve health, create peace and a harmonious relationship.
Vastu Shastra is a traditional space design system from India that aims to integrate architecture with nature, the relative functions of various parts of the structure, and ancient beliefs utilising geometric patterns (yantra), symmetry, and directional alignments. Vastu is derived from the word Vasty meaning a place of dwelling and Shastra means science.

Ayurvedic books contain clear instructions to use Vastu Shastra while buildings hospitals, temples and other public places. This approach has been adopted in India for centuries. I have also personally used these principles of design both in my home and clinics, including the seating layout and colour co-ordination in line with Vastu Shastra teachings.

Ayurveda

Ayurveda (veda meaning knowdge or science, ayus meaning longevity) has an uninterrupted history of practice for over 3000 years. Ayurveda is known as the science of life and rooted in the knowledge revealed by ancient seers whose insights are compiled in the Vedas, the oldest texts of Hinduism. Vedas are the earliest forms of documented knowledge and practice.

Ayurveda underscores the commonalities observed in man and nature in order explain the human-life in totality. It starts by saying that every being is a blend of body, soul, mind and the 5 sense organs (ears, skin, eyes, tongue, and nose). The structural units of the human body are categorised and represented in Ayurveda in terms of doshas (bio, physic and chemical energies of the living body), dhatus (tissues) and malas (metabolic end products).

Health is defined as a state where in the dynamic balance of doshas, dhatus, and malas is maintained causing the metabolism to operate at optimum level and the mind, body, soul and sense organs assume a sublime position. Diseases are the manifestations of perturbations in the equilibrium of the body constitutes including doshas.

The objectives of Ayurveda are mainly twofold. The first being the maintenance of positive health and the other the treatment of diseases. On the basis of the objectives defined, the sum and substance of Ayurveda can be defined into two parts:
A healthy man's regimen – the maintenance of positive health (svasthavrttam) and the second - patients regimen

(aturavrttam), which deals with the curative and palliative measures employed for the medical and emotional care of the patient.

Ayurvedic massage

The Ayurvedic practice of abhyanga, or oil massage has many physical and mental benefits. The oils used are sesame oil, coconut oil, mustard or olive oil. This unique massage exhibits the following benefits:

- Stress relief
- Removal of fatigue
- Removes excess wind
- Improves vision
- Strengthens the body
- Increases longevity
- Induces sleep
- Strengthens the skin
- Improves skin coloud

Daily routines

- Walk at the most ideal times (in line with guidance from your practitioner)
- Empty your bowels and bladder immediately after the above
- Drink a glass of tepid water when waking up to encourage regularity
- Care for your mouth, teeth and tongue

Diet and Ayurveda

The act of eating, according to Ayurveda is akin to a sacred ritual, as it is important for the development our consciousness in addition to our physical health. When we eat, our stomach should be in a relaxed posture and should should be aware of the taste, texture and smell of the food. This will improve our digestion. One should also only drink warm water while eating.

Tips for Good digestion:

- Eat sitting down, in a settled environment
- Do not in front of the television or anything that distracts from the act of eating
- Do not not eat on the go or in a rush
- Eat breakfast before 8am and make lunch the biggest meal of the day
- Dinner should be light and early as eating too late can upset your digestive process.

Therapeutic Yoga

The yogic process of treatment comprises of three steps:

1. A proper diet
2. Adequate yoga practice with correct form
3. A good understanding of things which concern life as an individual.

The main principle to adhere to with regards to diet is to maintain a balanced and varied diet while eliminating those items from daily intake which are considered harmful.

This common recommended items of food for almost all patients are fruits, salads, leafy vegetables, green vegetables and pulses. For non-vegetarians, this can be supplemented with fish, lamb and chicken in moderation.

All diets should follow the same basic principles of eating which include:

- To eat slowly
- To eat only 85 per cent of the stomach's capacity
- To eat at least two hours before their retiring time at night
- To avoid food that is too hot and spicy or fried and roasted in abundance
- Consume tea or coffee in moderation

Yoga Practice

First thing in the morning, before breakfast is the best time to practice yoga. It can be done in the evening or any time provided the stomach is empty. The general rule is to give an interval of three to four hours after eating and then do yoga. One should try to practice yoga at the same time every day.

Medical manipulation

Osteopathy is a system of healing which is based on the principal theme hat mechanical and structural abnormalities adversely affect the harmony and efficiency of the body. When the spine is manipulated, the principal goal is to remove any mechanical hindrance to the restoration of natural movements in the affected joints. This is because an imperfectly functioning structure predisposes disease. Imperfect function in the joints also moisten the spinal column because of the proximity to the spinal cord and the spinal nerves. If vital structures are adversely affected by faulty and impaired mechanisms, then a disease may ensue.

Chronic cases may require psychotherapy and also joint injections.

Astrology

Most Hindus will have a horoscope made a few days after they are born. They consult an astrologer regularly during their lifetime and still use horoscopes to determine if a potential spouse is a good match and when is an auspicious time to have the wedding, especially in India. Astrology also states that if a couple are in love, then there is no need to match their horoscopes since they already have had a meeting of the mind.

If someone is going to have a major operation then it is wise to consult an astrologer. They will advise when the best time is to have this. This is common in India and a health minister, Mr Shanmuadas campaigned to have astrologers in hospitals. Planetary alignment and forces influence our lives as we all occupy the same universe and are subject to natural forces beyond our control.

Gem Therapy

The art of using gems and stones for Ayurvedic treatment and astrological purposes has existed in India for over 7000 years. Vedic astrology has clear guidelines on the use of gems for curing diseases and sorrows that plague humans due to the ill effects of the planets' malevolent positions. Navratna denotes the majestic combination of 'nine auspicious gemstones'. This comes from the Sanskrit word referring to nine gems, which represent the nine major planets of our solar system.

Unani: The Science of Graeco-Arabic medicine

This age-old art of healing has a history of medical science in ancient Greece and traces its subsequent journey into the Arab world of the 8th century, which saw the birth of a new system called Unami. This deals with the concept of the body, its humoral balance and the basic factors which cause disease in a manner which is both simple and precise.

This system of medicine was laid down by Greek philosophers and physicians including Hippocrates (460 BC) and Galen (131 AD). The Arabs then introduced this system to India in the 12th century. Hakim Abdul Hameed helped to advance the system in India and was awarded one of the highest awards of the Indian government, the Padma Bhushan. Unani medicine emphasises the power of self-preservation in order to maintain the correct humoural balance in the body, a pre-requisite for health.

Other Modes of Therapy

Exercise, Massage, Steam bath, Fomentation, Emesis, Purgation, Enema and diet.

The Advantages of Alternative Medicines

Alternative medicines apply an approach which encompasses the effects of lifestyle, environment and emotional wellbeing. It emphasises prevention of disease and self-care as opposed to treatment of symptoms. It also highlights connections between the body and mind. Psychological pressures can contribute all sorts of ailments including everyday viral infections such as the common cold. Researches provides cues that the immune system is in constant dialogue with the brain. Psychological difficulties can have a direct effect on how our immune systems respond to threats. This explains why people often fall ill when they find themselves called to occupy a new symbolic place: a death, a birth, a marriage and retirement etc. Even hearing bad news can exacerbate auto immune disorders.

These psychosomatic illnesses are due to the derangement between the body and the mind.

The rising of technology and IT systems within general practices means that the doctors are often inputting data while seeing the patients, with no eye contact. The human connection is gone and one is not allowed to interrupt the process. Today, doctors have to cope with a staggering amount of bureaucracy on top of their work-load resulting in less time to listen to patients or talk through their symptoms. A patient's biography, details of life events, aspirations or any challenges they may facing are all left by the wayside resulting in increased anxiety and mental stress for the one seeking help. This would indicate that a patient's symptoms actually get worse after seeing a doctor!

In addition to this, the limited and localised knowledge of super specialists in medicine as well as the reduction of the body to the sum of its parts has other consequences which could exasperate a patient's symptoms.

Hippocratic oath

- Respect and support their teachers
- Share medical knowledge with others who are interested.
- Use the knowledge of medicine and diet to help patients
- Avoid harming patients, including providing no "deadly medicine" even if requested to do so
- Avoid providing a "remedy" that causes abortion
- Seek help from other physicians when necessary
- Avoid "mischief" and sexual relationships with the patient
- Retain patient confidentiality

Integrated medicine

In any integrated medicinal clinic, the first person encountered is usually a skilled diagnostician and generalist who directs the patient to the most appropriate treatment. They will usually provide an initial treatment plan of the regimen therapy.

Medical hypnosis

Hypnosis has many benefits including for the relief of:

- Pains
- Stress
- Asthma
- Insomnia
- Phobia
- Addiction
- Mental shock

Tissue Salts

Tissue salts, also called cell salts or biochemical salts, are minerals and the same as those found in the earth's rocks and soils. These minerals should be present in our bodies in a perfect balance, which is the prerequisite for complete health and well-being.
Dr.Schuessler (1828-1898) was an eminent 19th century German physician who discovered upon analysis, that when the human cell is reduced to ashes, it exhibits 12 minerals. He named this system biochemistry (the biochemistry of life) from the Greek word bios meaning " the course of life " and chemistry which means the knowledge of elements and the laws governing their nomination and behaviour .

The tissue salts should present in our food and are often found in those foods which have been grown organically in mineral-rich soils. In modern-day agricultural practices, soils are leached and life-sustaining minerals are boosted with chemicals fertilisers and fumigants. Tissue salts can be bought from every pharmacy and health shops.

The main tissue salts are:

- Cal fluor
- Cal phos
- Cal sulph
- Ferrum phos
- Kali mur
- Kali phos
- Mag phos
- Nat mur
- Nat phos
- Nat sup
- Silica

Health is the first prerequisite of all attainments in life. The attainment of health is not only an individual human aspiration but also a basic human right.

The World Health Organisation

Religion and medicine

Buddhism

Buddhism was founded around 2500 years ago in the North Eastern part of India by Siddartha Gautama who became Buddha or the enlightened one. Buddhists are usually vegetarians. Abortion is discouraged and there is no restriction on the use of contraception.

Christianity

Some catholics find any form of contraception unacceptable and permanent tubal sterilisation is prohibited by the Catholic faith.

Hinduism

Hinduism is where Ayurvedic treatments originate from. Women are highly regarded and the status of the mother is the pinnacle of status. It is common for Hindus to adopt lactovegetarian diets and to avoid pork. Cardiovascular disease and diabetes are common due to the diets.

Islam

Muslims believe that all is determined by God and that the final messenger on earth was the Prophet Muhammad. Their code of living is known as the five pillars of Islam which involves praying five times a day, fasting during the month of Ramadan, giving money to the poor and making a lifetime pilgrimage to Mecca (the pilgrimage is known as Hajj). Culturally, female Muslims may prefer to be treated by a female physician and men by males.

Sikhism

The Sikh faith was founded in the 16th century by Guru Nanak. The faith encourages doing good. Physical evidence of belonging to the Sikh faith is denoted by the fife K's which are Kesh (uncut hair), Kara (a steel bracelet), Kanga (a wooden comb), Kachera (cotton underwear) and Kirpan (a steel sward. A same sex physician is usually preferred.

Traditional Chinese Medicine

Chinese medicine is generally based on the balance of hot and cold, yin and yang and harmony within the universe. The Acupuncture treatments are widely available and popular. In Chinese culture, it is mostly the senior male member will be decision maker.

Jehovah's Witness and other religions

Jehovah's Witness are prohibited from accepting blood transfusions. Seventh-day Adventists promote a healthy life style and sponsor healthcare centres based on wholeness and the healing of body, mind and spirit.

Dedication

This book is dedicated to my beloved mother Ammu, who comes from a family of Ayurveda physicians. She taught some basis of Ayurveda treatments and took her children to Ayurveda or Homeopathic physicians since a young age, inspiring me to follow suit. She introduced me to and taught about alternative medicine. May her soul find peace.

About the Author

Dr Mannath Kulangara Ramachandran is affectionately known as Dr Ram and was born in India. He wanted to study medicine since an early age but unfortunately he suffered from Haemophobia, a fear of seeing blood that caused him to faint. When he said he wanted to become a doctor, everyone fell about laughing. He still pursued a career in medicine and had the last laugh, becoming a well-respected doctor, practicing in the UK for over four decades.

After studying medicine in India and working there, he came to the UK and initially worked as a paediatrician before becoming a GP in Essex. He later worked as a Homeopathist at the Royal College Hospital and set up a private practice in Harley Street. He was also invited to St James Palace by the (then) Prince of Wales, Prince Charles who would go on to become King Charles in 2022.

Dr Mannath Ramachandran is married to Rema and has dedicated his life to the service of others.

www.ingramcontent.com/pod-product-compliance
Lightning Source LLC
LaVergne TN
LVHW020542160826
845677LV00015B/4161

* 9 7 9 8 3 6 2 7 8 0 3 4 0 *